My First Pregnancy

Information, Advice, and Tips for New Parent

Table of Contents

Chapter 3: Just Baby

Introduction

Congratulations on your purchase of *My First Pregnancy,* and thank you so much for choosing this book. It is an honor to be included in such an important and impactful time of your life. Information is our most powerful ally during these moments of intense transition.

My goal in the creation of this book was to offer a resource to new mothers. Your mind is ablaze with questions, and you deserve a tool that you can lean on, that will provide you answers. In this book, we want to make it easy for you to both find and understand the common curiosities of a first pregnancy.

This book is also meant to be a safe haven for your thoughts. I keep the scary clinical language to a minimum so that you are better able to grasp the information that you're being given. So many resources for pregnant women are riddled with cold and uncaring statistics. I want to bring you all the answers that you need, and I would like to do so in a way that puts the numbers in context.

Bringing a new life into the world is one of the most profound experiences that any human being can have. Birth is a mirror that allows for the observance of one soul within another. Your little one is precious, and you can protect them preemptively by doing everything you can to both inform yourself and ease your own mind of its doubts. Let this book be a light by which you begin your journey of knowledge through the world of parenthood. Allow me to guide you through these moments of uncertainty toward the light of maternal love on the other side.

Chapter 1: Food, Drink, and Baby

One of the first queries from any expectant mother is how drastically her daily routine needs to change in order to account for the tiny life that she is now growing inside herself. I want to address these concerns in their own respective sections so that the information is more digestible. It is also preferable that the reader is able to thumb to a particular chapter to better find the answer to any pressing questions.

Food and dietary changes are the most infamous adjustments when it comes to pregnancy. We are bombarded with rumors and gossip that are curated with the intention of shocking the listener. Genuine facts are peppered into these narratives, but it is difficult to discern the real from the embellished. The following chapter is going to cut through all this abstraction, to hand you the truth. Continue reading to discover the answer to that question that has been bouncing around in your mind. You may even find answers to questions that you haven't thought of just yet.

The Famous Coffee Conundrum

A common piece of knowledge about pregnancy is that it is imperative to avoid caffeine like it's a leper plague. Do you really need to steer clear of your favorite beverage completely, or should you be finding a balance? What's so bad about coffee, anyway?

As it turns out, caffeine is not *all* bad. Less than two hundred milligrams a day is not harmful to you or the baby. An average cup of coffee is six to eight ounces and has from sixty to one-hundred milligrams of caffeine in it. This means that you should limit yourself to two or fewer brews a day.

It is worth noting that not all coffee is uniformly the same. Some brands and brews are stronger and will push the limits of what is recommended. You should look out for words like "espresso," as this can denote a much more caffeinated experience. We all know that espresso is known for the kick that it gives. One shot of the bitter powerhouse can plow through your daily budget by fifty milligrams of caffeine.

For those that prefer tea, you are allowed to indulge a little more. On the low end, most tea has about thirty milligrams of caffeine per serving. These numbers also have the potential to vary a bit more than coffee, with stronger cups coming in at around seventy milligrams. Black tea is the most potent of these, capping out at ninety milligrams of caffeine in a strong cup.

The coffee allowance conversation quickly loses its shine when you consider that the drink is not our only source of caffeine. Soda, chocolate, and even some over the counter (migraine) medications can quickly eat away at the daily recommended limit. A theme that will present itself over and over in this chapter is a mindfulness of the food and drink that is consumed during pregnancy. These guidelines can seem daunting at first, but it will quickly become a habit to check the contents of products before purchase.

Why is Caffeine Dangerous?

When considering the risk associated with the ingestion of any substance while pregnant, it is important to remember that the mother is sharing her body's resources with the developing fetus. The life that is being formed inside the womb is essentially a helpless blank slate. This slate is to be painted with the colors of its' environment.

Can you remember the moment that your parents first allowed you to have a soda? Or the first time that you ever tried an energy drink? This story is likely accompanied by fond memories of a silly young you, bouncing off the walls. For most of us, drinking the same beverage today would not produce a reaction of identical intensity.

Tolerance (and the lack thereof) is a key player in these early memories. It is difficult to drink a cup of coffee that feels as though it doesn't touch our fatigue now and imagine that the young life within us is struggling to handle the same chemicals. The baby's metabolic processes are still forming, which has an impact on the way that their system interprets caffeine. It can cause restlessness and abnormal sleeping patterns.

There are many contrasting reports about the effects of caffeine on pregnancy. In this book, we are only going to examine the claims that are backed by evidence. The chemical can elevate the mother's heart rate and can potentially raise blood pressure. Caffeine is also a diuretic (meaning it leads to frequent urination), which can potentially dehydrate the mother. There are some studies to suggest that low birth weight can also result as a consequence of habitually high caffeine consumption. High, in this instance, is more than two-hundred milligrams daily.

Alcohol and Pregnancy

Alcohol is a tricky subject when it comes to pregnancy. Ale and wine are some of the oldest libations known to our species. The love of drink is something that seems almost ingrained in our DNA. This topic is also one of the most widely debated, even among doctors. Everyone has an opinion, but what exactly is the fact in all of this back and forth? To understand the answer clearly, it is necessary to cut through some of this ambiguity.

Our starting point should be a statement that every doctor will agree with. Heavy drinking while pregnant is dangerous. Heavy, in this instance, is three or more units per day. There is evidence that prolonged exposure to alcohol can cause serious brain damage in fetuses. Fetal Alcohol Syndrome is one of the most common and well-known examples of the adverse effects that large-scale consumption can lead to. There is also the potential for stillbirth, miscarriage, learning and mental disabilities, low birth weight, preterm birth, and delivery complications. Binge and heavy drinking during pregnancy are highly risky. Those with alcohol addictions should seek help quickly, in order to safely wean themselves off for at least the length of gestation.

The rule of thumb is that heavy alcohol use within the first three months of pregnancy can affect the baby while it is still in the womb (miscarriage, delivery issues, premature birth, and low weight); while drinking after the first three months is more likely to result in Fetal Alcohol Syndrome or developmental and behavioral abnormalities later down the road. Alcohol is a toxin and will work against the growing baby. It can chemically alter or destroy the fetus's cells. The way in which it affects the baby is dependent upon the areas in which the fetus is developing when the substance is consumed.

Light and moderate drinking is a fuzzy area. Some doctors state with confidence that a glass of wine a day does not have an impact on the growing fetus. The issue with the statement is that the line is thin, and everybody is different. Moderation is always advised, and one should never drink until they are intoxicated (while pregnant).

Other doctors state that the only way to completely protect one's self is to abstain. Given the severity of the consequences, this is probably the wisest choice. When push comes to shove, pregnancy is only nine months. It is easy to replace alcohol with other means of relaxation; music, sex, meditation, baths, writing, reading, and drawing are just a few options. Order a virgin drink when out with friends and allow yourself to soak in the moments spent with those you love.

Most people, though, will find a place in between light drinking and total abstinence, and that is completely fine. Having a glass of wine every now and then is not linked to developmental issues. Allowing yourself to indulge only on special occasions is much easier than trying to change your entire routine or depriving yourself completely. This is not daily drinking. This is having a beer at your friend's birthday party or sipping wine on New Year's. This is the place where most of the population falls on this issue.

What If I Drank Before I Knew?

Having several drinks on a few occasions very early in the pregnancy is not linked to developmental damage. Everything will be just fine as long as the expectant mother quells her thirst after receiving the news that she is pregnant. Our bodies tend to forgive us for the occasional misdeed, provided we are not being habitually destructive.

Is Food Cooked with Alcohol Safe to Eat while Pregnant?

Alcohol has been used in food for as long as the libation has been available. Wine, liquor, and beer are added to some dishes to provide an interesting depth of flavor. Should you be as concerned about consuming alcohol in prepared meals, as you are about consuming the drinks themselves?

The answer to this question is also highly dependent. The simplest course of action would be to avoid food prepared with alcohol, just to be safe. Abstaining from the things we love can be complicated, though, and luckily this is not a cut and dry scenario.

Extended cooking has the potential to burn off the alcohol that you want to avoid. If the dish has been heated for two and a half hours, then less than five percent of the original alcohol remains. There is also evidence to suggest that if a lid is left propped up while the dish is simmering, more alcohol will evaporate than if the lid is left closed. Adding water to a simmering pot will also assist in the dilution.

Cakes tend to cling to the alcohol more. Thus it is not recommended that you order any cake that is cooked with alcohol. Dishes (like Tiramisu) that have the drink added after the food is cooked will not have a change in the acholic content. Food that is cooked for fifteen minutes or less will retain around half of its alcoholic content.

Small and infrequent drinks during pregnancy are largely thought to be harmless. Abstinence will still be the trustworthy and foolproof method of protecting yourself from the harm of any substance. It is a personal choice for the mother, which route she wishes to take. The occasional meal that has been simmered in wine, beer, or liquor is not believed to be enough to cause developmental issues within the fetus.

Moderation is again the answer to this question. Some dishes are more heavy-handed with their preparation and should be avoided, just to be safe. When you eat out, it would be to your benefit to inquire with the server about the amount of alcohol in the meal that you're eyeing. Vodka sauce and penne may, unfortunately, have to wait until the baby has arrived, but the occasional foray into other areas of fancy Italian cuisine is completely understandable.

Deli Meats, Smoked Fish and Soft Cheese

Deli meat and soft cheese are a more complex issue. The hesitation of doctors to recommend the consumption of ready-to-eat foods stems from the inability to know with one-hundred-percent certainty what you are ingesting. Listeria is the villain behind these concerns as it has a particular affinity for pregnant women, young children, and the elderly. This is a bacterium that can cause serious infections in those that are most vulnerable to it.

Listeria commonly rears its ugly head in deli meats or food that contains unpasteurized dairy. On very rare occasions, the bacterium has made its way into fruit and vegetables. One of the more famous outbreaks occurred when contaminated cantaloupes were sold to the public, causing almost one-hundred and fifty people in the U.S to fall ill.

The bacteria can fester in fecal matter, water, and soil. When the manure that farmers use to fertilize their crops is contaminated, it can cause wide-spread damage. The facts about listeria can appear to be frightening to an expectant mother, but arming yourself with knowledge is your first defense against falling victim, yourself.

Keeping your refrigerator set low enough in temperature will discourage the growth of this bacteria. Forty-degrees Fahrenheit is the highest that doctors recommend you allow your refrigerator to go. Your freezer should be set to zero degrees Fahrenheit.

Being mindful of the foods that you consume will also assist in your ability to avoid this potential hazard. Studies have shown that drinking milk while pregnant can decrease the risk of your child being born with asthma. However, raw milk is a breeding ground for bacteria. Be sure that you are consuming milk that has been pasteurized, meaning that the impurities have been removed. Soft cheese is a risky snack for the same reason. Smoked fish is also susceptible to contamination, so it is best to be mindful of the way that seafood is cooked during your pregnancy. Deli meats can be vulnerable to infestation also, so it is advised to avoid these. Raw sprouts and greens can also be hazardous.

Should you find yourself craving deli meats, cook them. Properly heating up food is a great way to kill bacteria. The safest course of action is to abstain, but life is not always so simple. Steam is your indication that you have warmed your cold cuts enough to be safe from listeria. Hot dogs are safe as long as they are cooked until they are over one-hundred and sixty degrees (Fahrenheit).

The bottom line when it comes to listeria is that you will be safe as long as you take a moment to consider your food. Less than three hundred people a year (in the United States) die from contact with this contaminant. That can sound like a large number, but there are over three-hundred-million people in America right now. It is worth it to understand that you are at greater risk and must be slightly more intentional in your consumption of food. Knowing about the brands that you are buying and cooking everything you eat (even if only for the next nine months) will astronomically improve your chances when it comes to the risk of getting a bacterial infection.

Everything Fish

In the section above, we discussed one of the many reasons that it is advisable for pregnant women to consume meals that have been properly cooked and prepared. We also hear quite a lot about the dangers of eating sushi while pregnant. What if sushi were the exception, and you were allowed to indulge in the craving? The worry is that pregnant women could potentially ingest parasites from seafood and get an infection or fall victim to food poisoning.

I have some good news. The fish that is used in sushi is generally **salmon** that has been farmed and not wild-caught. This means that they were flash-frozen to preserve them on their way to the restaurant. Flash freezing kills off those nasty parasites and makes the meat safe to eat. Pregnant women are also allowed to partake in sushi made from cooked fish. Avoid shellfish until after the baby comes, as that is where the danger lies. The danger of becoming ill from a fish that doesn't live in a shell is one in two million.

Three (safe) fishy meals a week is shown to dramatically reduce the stress that an expectant mother may experience. This can be an absolutely invaluable tool to have in your arsenal when everything around you is determined to test your patience and coping skills. There is also evidence that eating the right fish can improve both your mental acuity and that of your unborn child.

Omega-3 fatty acids (fish oil) are the magic compound within fish that give it so many benefits to both mother and child. They are necessary nutrients for optimal body function and health. These fatty acids also do not occur on their own within humans, which means that it is imperative for us to incorporate them into our diets. We do a poor job of that in the west, according to nutritional scientists. This deficiency can be made worse for pregnant women because the baby uses up Omega-3s when building its nervous system. Benefits of fish oil for developing fetuses include increased cognitive function, visual responsiveness, increased birth weight, lowered chance of food allergies, and gastrointestinal health. The benefits of fish oil are immense and should be present in the mother's diet (either through fish or supplements) to encourage the healthy development of her child.

DHA (or docosahexaenoic acid) and EPA (or eicosapentaenoic acid) are types of omega-3 fats. The names are not important, but it is necessary to know that these abbreviations are associated with the two key omega-3 fats that pregnant women should be supplementing into their diets in some way. Should an expecting mother dislike the taste of fish or just be wary of the parasites (as discussed above) or mercury content (which will be addressed below), then she should be able to find a supplement with the label DHA and EPA to add to her daily routine.

There must still be some discretion about which fish you indulge in as an expecting mother. Parasites are not your only concern. Salmon is still one of the safest and tastiest options, and luckily it will remain on the approved table for this discussion.

Mercury also presents a danger to developing fetuses and may be found in higher levels in some fish. Tuna is famous for its toxin content and has been a hot topic of debate for many years. When it comes to canned tuna, light is safer than albacore. The FDA states that a pregnant woman may safely eat twelve ounces of lower mercury fish a week. Safe fish is as follows: salmon, catfish, canned light tuna, pollock, and fish sticks. Six ounces of albacore tuna, fresh tuna or locally caught fish are allowed. Stay away from sharks and other large fish until after the pregnancy.

Understanding Medication While Pregnant

There are so many comprehensive lists out there with the names of safe and unsafe medications to take while pregnant. There is also no one more knowledgeable about your particular needs, than your doctor. Trust your doctor before you trust these conflicting lists compiled from the internet because the advice you receive will be more tailored to you as an individual. It is still helpful to be armed with the knowledge of the ways that pregnancy can alter your medication because, again, knowledge is our weapon against unnecessary stress.

Pregnancy alters the way that your body functions. More blood pumps at a greater pace through the kidneys (your filtration system). This means that your internal organs are working harder to care for the additional strain on your internal resources; because of these changes, substances that would normally remain in your system for long enough to effect change are being ushered out before they are able to fulfill their purpose. Your health provider may switch you from your normal medication to something that works more fluidly with your changing body.

The F.D.A mandates that all prescription medications have effects on pregnant mothers available on their label. Three sections address those concerns: the pregnancy, lactation and reproductive potential. Under each of these labels, there is information about how the medicine will affect a mother during the various stages of conception. The pregnancy summary will give the consumer an idea of the statistical likelihood of their child developing critical abnormalities from coming in contact with the substance. Lactation allows the mother an estimate of how much of the drug will be passed along through the mother's milk when she is breastfeeding.

This mountain of information can seem overwhelming and intricate, even without a deeper look inside the functions of medications while pregnant. Luckily, this is not something that needs to be added to the list of worries for any new mother. Bring a list of your medications to your general practitioner, including over-the-counter medications that you take with some frequency. Avoid aspirin and ibuprofen, Tylenol is okay should an emergency fever medication be needed. Staying hydrated is also a valuable way to fight illness and dehydration.

Antidepressants During Pregnancy

This small section about antidepressants is being added, even though it was just advised to speak to your doctor about all medications because that sentiment will send some expecting mothers into a panic. Antidepressants are necessary for the healthy function of a large portion of the population. Depression also has the potential to physically harm the growing fetus. There is good news, there are antidepressants (usually SSRIs) that have been shown to be low risk for unborn children and pregnant mothers. The doctor will generally find the safest chemical and dose for the individual with an emphasis on limiting the exposure for the fetus.

What about Prenatal Vitamins?

The words "prenatal vitamins" seem to be on the tip of everyone's tongue when you're expecting, but why are they necessary? Many assume that vitamins are recommended to stay at peak physical condition and that is why they are ideal for expecting mothers, but that isn't completely correct. We have seen a theme that will keep popping up throughout the more medical topics. The body of a pregnant woman is expending more energy than it is familiar with, to account for the new life growing within. A woman in the throes of gestation is rapidly depleting her stores of nutrients on her unborn child, which means that they must be replaced.

The amount of protein that is recommended to maintain health almost doubles during pregnancy. We have also covered the rapid depletion of omega-3 fatty acids, because of their function in building the nervous system of the fetus.

Herbal supplements are another beast entirely and they should be treated as medication. It is imperative that a pregnant mother relay her relationship with these supplements to her primary care provider as she would any other medication. To the surprise of many, most herbal supplements should be avoided during pregnancy.

Prenatal vitamins are a safe blend of many of the micronutrients that are necessary for the growth and health of both mother and child. Clinical evidence supports the use of these supplements with overwhelming evidence of a reduction of preterm birth and even preeclampsia.

Recommended pregnancy vitamins include folate, vitamin D, iron, magnesium, and calcium. Luckily, this can also be added to the list of things that need not be worried about. Prenatal vitamins include all these necessary nutritional supplements, meaning that picking a good prenatal vitamin can cross all of this off your list. Prenatal vitamin regimens should start when you are trying to conceive. Didn't know you were pregnant? That's okay too, just begin taking the supplements now with the knowledge that you have conquered another necessary task and you are doing great!

What is Folic Acid?

Your baby's brain and spinal cord are precious and important parts of their development, and they are formed within the first three months of pregnancy. Monitoring your intake of folic acid can safeguard against potential birth defects with both of these. Folic acid works to increase the amount of blood in your body, which is the lifeforce by which your baby is created. Prenatal vitamins include folic acid or folate to make it easier for expectant mothers to intake more of the nutrient.

It is a good idea to begin taking folic acid a month before you plan to conceive or from the moment that you're aware that you are pregnant to the first three months (400-800 micrograms a day). If you live in America, the FDA has stepped up to assist you in this department. Due to the number of unplanned pregnancies in the United States, the FDA has ensured that many of the foods that are consumed on a daily basis are fortified with folic acid. Cereal, pasta, and rice are all great sources for the essential nutrient.

Hydration and Water Intake

The general recommended amount of water consumption each day is widely known to be eight cups. During pregnancy, your intake will jump to **ten cups a day** on average. This has the potential to rise even more if you exercise or are just living in a hot climate.

Thirty-two percent of new mothers have issues with constipation, which may be addressed by increasing the amount of water consumed. Hemorrhoids, UTIs, and swelling may also be positively affected by improving hydration. The most simple way to assess hydration is to check the color of one's urine; it should be clear to pale yellow. The sensation of thirst should also be kept to a minimum if water intake is high enough.

It is best to avoid soda as often as possible. The caffeine will eat away at the daily budget that we have already discussed. Sugar from soft drinks can also contribute to health issues for mother and child.

Nutritional Changes

Previous sections have covered changes in micronutrients and the supplements that an expecting mother may use to stay on top of these needs. Now it is time to take a step back and look at the broader topic of general nutrition and how it evolves during gestation. What should you be eating to meet the changing needs of your body and the tiny life that you carry inside it?

The intensity of a mother's relationship to food will change right alongside nutritional needs. Expectant mothers know the real meaning of the word "hangry" and may experience some unexpected emotional responses to their body's new cravings. All of this is perfectly normal, and things will return to business as usual once the baby arrives.

Pregnancy Cravings

 can also be a telling clue to the nutrients that our body is asking us. Hormones can change the way that we perceive tasty treats, too, but sometimes our stomachs are trying to communicate to us in their own way. For instance, should your mouth water at the thought of a Starburst, it could mean that your body is begging for fruit but has botched the translation. Indulgence in the occasional carb or piece of candy is also a necessary part of keeping ourselves sane, but moderation is the magic word when it comes to appeasing the junk food cravings.

Pregnant women will often hear the phrase that they are "eating for two." The truth is, to support a pregnancy, it is only necessary to consume around three-hundred extra calories a day for the first trimester. This is, unfortunately, much less than a whole other person worth of meals. The amounts will increase slightly as pregnancy goes on to three hundred and forty extra calories in the second trimester and four-hundred and eighty in the third trimester. Mothers should expect to gain from fifteen to twenty-five pounds during pregnancy, according to nutritionists.

Major changes are necessary when it comes to the quality of our food, though. Those of us who eat in a more average than healthy way will feel the brunt of this shift. The developing a baby inside of a womb will leach away nutrients from mom, meaning that she must work more diligently to replace her vital reserves.

Ideally, a pregnant mother is meant to consume a healthy diet. She requires a variety of foods and meals that include both fruits and vegetables. Fish (as discussed in an earlier section) is also highly recommended for pregnant women. Fiber, calcium, zinc, and folate (synthetic folic acid) are also an important part of a new mother's diet.

Calcium and Calcium vs. Lactose

For expectant mothers, healthy dairy is a wonderful source of calcium. Yogurt is a perfect pregnancy food because it also comes packed with probiotics, which promote digestive health. It is important to remember that all dairy must be pasteurized, or it could potentially be more hazardous than helpful. Avoid raw milk and soft cheeses.

One of the many anomalies of the human body is the changes that a woman experiences during pregnancy and at the moment of childbirth. The process of creating another human life seems to inspire some creative tricks from within. For instance, the ability to produce lactose increases and continues to do so the later an expecting mother is into her pregnancy. This means that even a lactose intolerant individual may find themselves able to process milk and dairy with no issue.

There are other options available for women who can't or simply don't enjoy processing lactose. Other calcium-rich foods include broccoli, chickpeas, spinach, pinto beans, and tofu. There are also options like calcium-fortified almond milk.

Can I still Eat Honey?

Honey is everyone's favorite sweetener, but is it bad for babies? Turns out that honey is only harmful when given to an actual infant. You may continue to use the nectar while pregnant with no harm to you or your baby. Honey is sometimes pasteurized to prevent fermentation, but this has no bearing on it being risky.

One More Thing

In this chapter, we have explored everything that should and should not be consumed during one's pregnancy. I hope that you can use this section as a resource that you may return to, whenever you need the information. I hope that learning about the conditions behind the rules has allowed you to better understand where the guidelines originate from and the way in which your body reacts to change.

The human body is a marvelous contraption that adapts to almost anything you throw at it.

Women are capable of ushering new life into this world. Just think of all the beautiful and awe-inspiring things that you accomplish. Nutrients are just another brush for you to paint with. If you are careful and you make slow and intentional strokes, your masterpiece will reflect your care. If you hesitate or mess up a line every now and then, your work will still be brilliant and beautiful. One or two missteps do not ruin anything in the grand scheme of things. Trying your best to make the most ideal choices for your unborn child is the only thing that matters. Creatively faltering is something that just goes along with parenthood.

It should be made clear that guidelines are only there to illuminate the healthiest course of action. If/when you fail to ingest the right amount of fiber, the next time that you reach for a slice of pizza instead of broccoli or when you break down and have a small glass of wine with dinner, just know that it is okay to forgive yourself and move along. That is a sentiment that I would like for you to keep in mind as we continue through this book, as we will be discussing lifestyle changes and answering pregnancy's most burning questions.

Chapter 2: Lifestyle and Baby

This chapter will be devoted to taking a closer look at the way your daily activities change when you become pregnant. Work-life, exercise, weight gain, and many other topics will be brought to light. This book endeavors to cut through the conflicting information that new mothers are bombarded with in every direction. *Lifestyle and Baby* will paint a clear picture of the recommended adjustments that you can make to your routine in order to create the most ideal environment for the growing child inside you.

Working while Pregnant

Unfortunately, there is no one-size-fits-all answer for how long a mother should work into her pregnancy. Sometimes financial needs must be met, and other people are just bored when they are allowed too much time to sit with their own thoughts. Some women are too uncomfortable within their last trimester to continue showing up at a job every day. Expecting mothers will often try to stay active in the workforce until the very last minute so that they are free to spend their maternity leave with the newest addition to the family. None of these answers are wrong.

When you are deciding what is right for you, you must take into consideration how you feel. It is much easier to commit to being active when you aren't physically uncomfortable. High-risk pregnancies are also often advised to slow down in order to protect the baby. When picking your last day at work, it is helpful to assess how you have been handling your pregnancy thus far. This seems like a simple and silly point to make, but women are tough and will sometimes try to power through hard situations to spite their body warning them to take a step back. It can also be beneficial for an expecting mother to set aside a week or two to focus on herself before the baby arrives. This can drastically improve stress levels.

Legal Stuff

In America and around the world, there are laws put into place that protect new mothers from discriminatory businesses. **The Pregnancy Discrimination Act** asserts that employers must treat pregnancy as a temporary disability. This allows for the same time off and reinstatement privileges that are given to others with temporary disabilities.

The Family and Medical Leave Act (or FMLA) requires that employers with more than fifty employees (that work within seventy-five miles of the business) allow up to twelve weeks of medical leave for maternity. Thirty days' notice must be provided to the employer, and the mother may be asked to provide proof of the pregnancy from a doctor. For the mother to be in the protected class of this act, she must have worked with the company for more than one year. She is also required to have worked 1,250 hours over the course of the year.

FMLA also assures the expecting mother that she is allowed to return to her job when her maternity leave is over. Her benefits may not be taken away from her, while she is away on leave. The employer is not allowed to treat maternity leave as an unexcused absence.

Tips for Working while Expecting

Working while your body is trying to grow a new life inside of it can be a hassle. Sometimes it will seem as though your whole system is working against you. It will frustrate you that you are not able to complete tasks that you used to breeze through. These are the moments that you must summon your strength and remember that you roll with the punches. The following tips will make it easier to fight back against the discomfort.

Avoid the breakroom or any other food-related areas that could potentially inundate you will strong smells. This is especially true if you have been suffering from nausea on a daily basis. Close your eyes now and picture your workplace. Are there any other areas that act as an assault on the senses? Because avoid those places too.

Do not tell coworkers your baby's name until after the birth. People are thoughtless and silly sometimes, and expecting mothers are already trying to handle thirty other things. It can be a bad idea to add coworker Jim's opinion of your child's name to that list.

Take breaks and do not be ashamed to do so. Your body needs every ounce of rest that it can achieve. This means finding meaningful rest at home too and sleeping for a full eight hours.

Snack on healthy foods throughout the day. This will help with your energy levels, which will be dropping more than ever. Water can also be a creative means of keeping one's self awake. Hydration should be a goal in general, so adding some extra water to your workday is a good idea all around.

Wear comfortable clothes and shoes in the workplace. As time progresses and your pregnancy advances, discomfort is going to become more and more of a daily obstacle. You can combat this by ensuring that you are changing positions and wearing clothes that are not restrictive. This goes right along with taking breaks because standing up or walking around can also work to reduce fluid buildup.

Find a support network within your job. People will always tell you that it isn't a good idea to make friends at work, but we have learned that sometimes people can be wrong. The last thing that you need is a room full of people who make you feel isolated. You will be going through some hormonal changes and some intense discomfort from time to time. Talking to your coworkers will lift some of that despondency off of your shoulders and will also open you up to receiving help when it is available.

This last tip is going to be an obvious one but stay away from ladders. Do not pick up anything heavy. Do not place yourself in a position of personal risk. Avoid cleaning or being around any harsh chemicals.

The Dreaded Litterbox

Speaking of harmful chemicals, it is time to address the weirdest piece of advice about pregnancy that many of us have ever heard. The reason that expecting mothers are told to leave the litterbox to someone else is the risk of toxoplasmosis. Toxoplasmosis is an infection caused by a parasite that lives in the gut and fecal matter of housecats. This is another one of those infections that prefers pregnant women and those with otherwise weakened immune systems. This infection is given to humans upon the accidental ingestion of feline fecal matter.

When at all possible, leave the litterbox cleaning to someone else. If it becomes absolutely necessary for you to take on the task, gloves and thoroughly washing your hands will greatly reduce your risk of catching the infection. The good news is, the danger is limited to the litterbox. The offending parasite is not able to live on your cat's fur, so there is no danger in otherwise cuddling up to your pet.

Exercising while Pregnant

Most exercise is both safe and recommended during pregnancy. Strenuous exercise should be avoided, but light and moderate movement is ideal. This section is going to focus more on keeping up with your existing routine. If you were active before you became pregnant, then you will be able to remain active after. In fact, exercise can help with many of the aches and pains that tend to accompany a progressing pregnancy.

Pregnancy is not the most ideal time to try and pick up a new exercise routine. Walking, swimming, and stationary bikes are the safest activities. Low impact is a good phrase to keep in

mind when trying to rearrange your workout
session to protect your little one.

Pregnancy and Travel

Traveling while pregnant can sometimes be
unavoidable, but is it safe? As it turns out, the
safe to travel up until the thirty-sixth week of
your gestation. Many airlines will allow
expecting mothers to fly until the thirty-sixth
week, with some international airports only
permitting travel until the twenty-eighth week.
The second trimester is the most comfortable
and risk-free time during which to traverse long
distances.

During the first trimester, morning sickness can
prove to be a hindrance to your plans. Airplanes
and buses can add motion sickness on top of a
growing list of nausea issues. The third trimester
can prove to make travel difficult because there
is always a possibility that your plans may
become derailed by labor.

With the ability to travel comes an assumed
responsibility on the mother's part. It is a good
idea to schedule an appointment with your
primary care provider to assess if the trip is a
good idea. Doctors will be more able to answer
these questions for the individual, as they are
able to take into account all aspects of the
pregnancy thus far. Vaccines are also an

important consideration when travel is imminent. It's also a good idea to form loose plans that can easily be adjusted if an issue were to arise. Bring your approved over-the-counter medications to aid with gas and nausea. Ginger can be a safe herbal supplement to aid in motion sickness. Hydration is also important, so if you should find yourself in a plane while pregnant, be sure to drink plenty of water.

Sex

Pregnancy hormones can cause an increase in libido that can leave some expecting mothers wondering if sex is still on the table. The good news is that sex is completely safe until the last weeks of pregnancy. Those that fear for the baby's physical safety will be pleased to know that the developing fetus is secure behind a wall of the uterine muscle. The amniotic sac also acts as a cushion that protects the developing baby. The spasms that your body experiences during orgasm have nothing to do with the contractions that you will feel in labor, so you may engage in sex guilt-free.

There are some instances when sexual activity is recommended to cease, but this is primarily only an issue for pregnancies that are already high-risk. If you are carrying twins, then your pregnancy is already considered delicate, and sex should be avoided until birth. Mothers who have been warned by their doctors about the risk of miscarriage or pre-term birth will also be advised to abstain from penetration until the baby has been safely delivered. Vaginal bleeding, discharge or cramping that occurs for no known reason, should be addressed with a doctor. Sex should be avoided until the mother has received advice from a medical professional.

Sunlight

Pregnancy hormones change the way that the body reacts to sunlight. It is much easier to achieve a sunburn if you're expecting. It is also much easier to find your skin discolored by time spent outdoors.

Worse than discoloration and burning, though, is the fact that a pregnant woman's risk of developing skin cancer also increases. The best way to protect one's self is to avoid the sun. Should you have to venture outside, wear at least 30 SPF sunscreen and a nice big hat.

Body and Skin during Pregnancy

The way that pregnancy is portrayed on the silver screen can be misleading. According to Hollywood, women are supposed to glow when pregnant. Should you happen to not be a lightning bug or one of the fortunate few, this section is for you. We will be discussing the more realistic changes that occur within the human body during gestation.

The most common change to a women's skin during pregnancy is a darkening of pigmentation. Skin that is naturally slightly more shaded before will be more pronounced and pigmented after a woman conceives. Examples of the areas that may be affected: underarms, nipples, skin around the belly button, inner thighs and undereye, etc., Dark spots will also form on the faces of around seventy percent of pregnant women, making it **very important** to wear broad-spectrum sunscreen and protect one's skin. Pigmentation will often return to normal in the months following the birth, but dark spots caused by the sun can potentially be permanent. Find a good sunscreen and avoid direct contact with sunlight whenever possible. Hats can also be helpful. Half of the pregnant women will also experience white splotches around their forehead.

Moles have a tendency to morph and change during pregnancy. This can be an issue for some women because it is difficult to discern the difference between a pregnancy-related change and a more serious change in moles. If you are prone to freckles and/or moles, it is imperative that you keep an eye on your skin during pregnancy. Should you notice discoloration, a change in size or symmetry, or any other shift in appearance, it's important that you bring this information to a doctor immediately.

Some of the less frightening bodily ailments include varicose veins and redness of the hands. Gums will also be very quick to bleed during pregnancy, which can make flossing more of a challenge. Swelling in the lower half of the body occurs because the developing fetus has the potential to block flowing blood from returning to the upper half. This is a normal occurrence and is not troubling unless the swelling occurs in the face and persists into the last trimester.

One of the more grisly looking (but completely harmless) side-effects of pregnancy is something called a pyogenic granuloma. These manifest as open, leaking sores. They will ooze blood or puss. Pyogenic granulomas look like an emergency, but they are common and not cause for concern. They are shiny lumps that are, on average, around the same size as the tip of a thumb and present as raw flesh. These are referred to as "pregnancy tumors," but don't let the name scare you. They are easily removed, and often go away on their own, as soon as the baby is delivered. These unfortunate lesions have a tendency to pop up on hands and inside mouths.

Stretch marks

Stretch marks are a natural part of pregnancy that affects some women more drastically. This is an unavoidable part of the process with ninety percent of pregnant women experiencing the scars. Stretch marks are formed when weight is gained rapidly and the elastin in our skin is stressed to the point of snapping. The far less headache-inducing way to deal with these is to accept them. Accepting can be easier said than done, though, and there are a few advancements that make reducing stretchmarks an attainable goal.

This is such common stress that companies have jumped on the opportunity to make money from "miracle cures." It doesn't matter as much what you use, as long as you heavily moisturize the areas that are most likely to stretch (stomach, breasts, lower back and hips) before the stretching begins. Vitamin E, shea butter, and cocoa butter are all great ingredients to look out for in a moisturizer. This will increase the strength of the elastin in your skin so that it can take more of a hit when things begin to expand. Burt's Bees Mama Bee Belly Butter is a good starting point, should you feel lost on choosing a moisturizer.

Stretch mark damage can also be mitigated by monitoring your weight gain. Increasing your body weight slowly can help immensely when it comes to your skin. Scars are easiest to treat when they are fresh. This means that moisturizing while they are still pink can provide the best results. When a scar has faded back into your skin tone, it can be impossible to change.

There is also one FDA approved laser treatment that claims to improve the look of the marks by fifty to seventy-five percent; it's called Laser Stretch Mark Removal. It is the most effective manner to repair the scars, but it is also the most side-effect heavy. The skin will be raw and scabbed after treatment, and each treatment costs around three thousand dollars, with many additional fees for consultation, follow-ups, etc. The patient will have to avoid strenuous activity and be very careful about the sun protection after the session. The laser works by simulating damage to the skin tissue (while the client is numbed), to which the body responds with collagen to the site of the scars. Over time, this can drastically improve the look of the marks.

There is no evidence that moisturizers can heal stretch marks after-the-fact. Watch out for any lotions that claim to make the scars disappear. With this statement in mind, there are a few doctor-recommended methods that are far less expensive and traumatic than laser treatments. The most practical is to invest in an exfoliant to clear away the dead skin from the affected areas. Follow this up with an anti-aging moisturizer with retinol that promotes collagen production.

Please note: any moisturizer with retinol should have an opaque bottle that shields it from the elements, as retinol loses its effectiveness (oxidizes) when exposed to light and air. Do not buy any clear bottles or jars that boast about containing retinol, because it will be rendered useless.

Acne

Acne is another very common issue for pregnant women. There are also skin reactions that mimic acne well enough to convince some ladies that they are suffering from something that isn't actually affecting them. Addressing this faux acne first, body chemistry changes when carrying a child. During the length of the pregnancy, some women become allergic to substances that never caused an issue before. Should you notice that your acne is closer to your hairline than your t-zone, it is likely that you have developed an allergy to your shampoo or conditioner. Switching to new products should eliminate skin irritation. The new shampoo should be clear.

Half of all pregnant women will experience acne due to a change in hormones. Hormones control the level of oil that our skin produces. Being prone to pregnancy acne has a lot to do with genetics, and a good indication that you will have bouts of breakouts is if your skin reacted similarly during your period. Surprisingly, the increase in oil production is what gives some women the famous "pregnancy glow."

Handling acne during pregnancy can be a pain because many of the most effective prescription medications could potentially damage the fetus. The safest and most efficient ways to manage your breakouts include:

- Wash your face once in the morning and once at night.
- Make sure that your own hands and other objects do not touch your face. Every time your skin comes in contact with another surface, there is a potential for bacteria to spread.
- Change your pillowcase with frequency.
- Be sure that you are not over-cleaning your face.

Weight Gain

Pregnant women should be gaining anywhere from twenty-five to thirty-five pounds over the course of the pregnancy. This number can shift based upon the pre-pregnancy weight of the mother. Smaller women need to gain more weight for their gestation; larger women need to gain less. The average expecting mother needs to gain around three pounds during the first three months of pregnancy. After the first trimester, she should gain one pound a week.

Most pregnancy weight will be lost after the birth of the child. Twenty percent of women will hold on to the extra pounds, finding it more difficult to drop back to their pre-pregnancy weight. The majority of women will retain less than ten pounds of extra weight for their first year after being pregnant.

If these numbers are terrifying, and you have already blown through the amount of weight that you were supposed to gain during your pregnancy, you are not alone. Nearly half of the pregnant women in the U.S have gained more than the advised amount of weight. What are the consequences of that extra weight?

The CDC warns that both too much pregnancy weight and not enough are both dangerous. There is a chance that the baby could grow to experience childhood obesity when they have come from a mother whose weight was higher than it was supposed to be. More weight can also make it more difficult to lose the pregnancy pounds after the child is born. There are also some known links to high blood pressure and other complications, but a recent study is causing medical professionals to question this.

There is evidence that if a mother was already overweight, then gaining more weight than recommended doesn't change her risk of complication. Doctors still suggest that mothers attempt to monitor and control their weight, but the connection from pounds gaining during pregnancy and birth complications is not as strong as previously thought.

Exercise and diet can be an important ally in keeping pregnancy weight under control. Doctors suggest that a pregnant woman should be physically active for at least one hundred and fifty minutes a week. Ensuring that the mother's diet is full of fruits, vegetables, and food with nutritional value can make the pregnancy much easier and more comfortable to navigate.

Stress and How to Manage

Stress is, unfortunately, another natural side-effect of pregnancy. There is so much planning, worry, and doubt that goes into creating another human life. There are many sleepless nights and small medical emergencies; the process is enough to wind-up even the most mellow among us. The insidious aspect of stress is that it produces more stress, as pregnant mothers are concerned that the anxiety will harm the baby.

The good news is that stress on its own, can not hurt the baby. As long as the mother stays consistent with sleep and nutrition, the fetus will be safe. Coping with stress in negative ways is where things get tricky. It is important for your own mental health, to find ways to manage the stress. Speaking to your medical professional is the first step toward mitigating the symptoms of stress.

Meditation and meditative breathing have a rich history of helping with these issues. It is important for the mother to find time for herself, which is why hobbies can also provide some relief. There are yoga classes that are geared exclusively toward pregnant women, offering many of the best parts of meditation with the added benefit of maintaining flexibility. For those that get frustrated and wound-up in a physical way and need that release of tension, exercise is a wonderful way to keep one's self level-headed. Warm (not hot) baths can help with both physical and mental overstimulation, light a candle, lean back in the tub and relax.

Stress can also be handled by taking control of the situation. Planning is a huge part of this control, and creating a birth plan will eliminate a lot of uncertainty. If you are concerned about money, write down your expenses and prioritize the most important. Should you be concerned about the actual delivery, watch videos and read testimonies about women who have had very positive experiences. Share these activities with your partner, a friend or family member. Allow for a conversation to take place, one where you are very open and honest about your feelings.

Maternity Shoes

As the pregnancy progresses, there is more and more strain on women's feet. The physical shifts in her body mean that the distribution of her weight is different than it has ever been before. The fetal roadblock in her abdomen means that the lower half of her body is swollen and uncomfortable. Sudden extra weight means that her feet and prior shoes have both taken a beating.

Keep one of the most important parts of your body and your means of mobility, pleased. For your own sanity. Mothers should purchase some flat, cushioned and breathable shoes with extra room. The best pregnancy footwear is comfortable sandals and slip-on tennis shoes with memory foam insoles.

Avoid Avoid Avoid

The long list of things to avoid can be overwhelming when you're pregnant. Most deodorants are off-limits, a good portion of hair products with silicone are off-limits, paint, bleach, the litterbox, etc., Pregnant women should avoid ladders, strenuous chores, and chemical cleaners. Should you have no choice but to clean, open a window, and use thick latex gloves. If you are a smoker, then now is the time to quit.

Amazon has a useful feature in the search. You may type in *pregnancy safe shampoos, pregnancy-safe conditioners, pregnancy-safe skincare, pregnancy-safe deodorant,* and more. Shopping online can allow you to cut through having to learn giant lists of products that you are or are not allowed to use. For shampoos and conditioners, you are looking for something that is sulfate, silicone and paraben-free. Most safe shampoos will advertise on their labels if they do not include these ingredients.

Deodorants need to be free of aluminum, which most natural deodorants will also advertise. There is a good deal of skincare products that become off-limits when you become pregnant, including anything with salicylic acid. Sunscreen even needs to be natural, according to some dermatologists. Most acne-fighting ingredients are toxic to a growing fetus, and BPA in the bottles of products can also be a contaminant.

Should You create a Birth Plan?

Authoring a birth plan has some very apparent benefits but it can also be a way to handle anxiety related to the delivery of your child. A birth plan is essentially a list of preferences that a pregnant woman will create to hand out to anyone who will play a part in the delivery. It allows you to have a clear say in the way that you would like the birth handled, even if you are not able to articulate these desires when the day comes.

Birth plans are a wonderful idea for expecting mothers. They offer a perfect chance to ease her mind about the uncertainty of delivery. Once the labor starts and chaos ensues, it's easy to be pushed forward through the events of the day. With a birth plan, a more level-headed you from months ago has taken care of asserting all of your needs to family, friends, and medical staff. Templates are easy to find online so that you don't even have to worry about brainstorming the queries. Birthing plans will address some of the following (for example):

- Who will be present?
- Is there a position in which the pregnant woman would prefer to give birth?
- Will there be skin to skin contact right away?
- Pain medicine preference.
- What else will be done for pain?
- Will the mother breastfeed right after birth?

These are just a small sample of the many items in a birth plan. Some health care providers will not be open to these kinds of preferences, but others will be more than willing to accommodate the patient. You also have the ability to schedule a meeting with the Labor and Birth Dept at your hospital of choice, to review your plan and make any necessary changes.

Birthing Class

There are so many activities that expecting mothers are expected to participate in. Is a birthing class worth your time and money? What can you expect from these classes? Why go to a place when you have the internet, and you can just research things at home?

A long time ago, birthing classes were not optional. In order for the doctors to allow your partner into the delivery room with you, you would have to complete a class and present proof. These classes are no longer a mandatory activity, but they are still very much worth a new mother's time. Women aim to take these classes during the second trimester.

Most insurance will cover the cost of birthing classes, which can range anywhere from fifty to two hundred dollars. They are available through the hospital, private educators and birthing centers. For the stay-at-home-and-research types, there are even birthing classes online. This book has done its best to make it clear that knowledge can vanquish uncertainty and doubt. These courses will ensure that you understand every step of the delivery process. There is even emphasis on making the correct choice for yourself and your child in the event of an emergency. The material that these instructors cover is invaluable to any expecting mother. Birthing classes also provide an opportunity to sit in front of a professional in childbirth with pen in hand. It is the perfect opportunity to ask questions and soak in probable years of expertise in labor and delivery. This is also a chance to bring your partner into the birthing fold with an experience that also serves to teach them how to be the best assistant that they can be when the day comes. Classes like this will allow your partner to understand their role in the delivery.

Knowledge is important. This book will hammer this point home as many times as it gets the chance, but it's a true statement for more than one reason. Stress immediately takes a nosedive when our anxieties are demystified. Birthing classes are a spotlight shining upon the dark and frightening world of labor and its freaky depiction in Hollywood movies. The course is also an interactive way to learn about the choices that you have concerning your labor, including natural birth, water birth, and many more. It is also a fun way to meet other women who are due around the same time that you are, which is the perfect excuse to make a new friend.

Preparing for Trouble

Postpartum depression is a dark reality for some new mothers. The thought that your brain chemistry could condemn you to feel hopeless during what should be the happiest moments of your life is frightening. The inability to get a full night's rest can compound on top of your body's unstable hormones to create an emotional storm. Men are also capable of experiencing this phenomenon.

Postpartum depression can include panic attacks, thoughts of worthlessness, isolation, inability to eat, and even difficulty bonding with your new baby. Thoughts of hurting yourself or the child are not uncommon. It starts a few days after the birth and may last as long as a couple of months. This is a dark topic in an otherwise hopeful book, so you may be asking yourself why we are covering it.

It is imperative that should you find yourself in the throes of postpartum sadness, its less intense brother *Baby Blues* or even the more severe postpartum psychosis, you understand that it isn't your fault. It is a birth complication and nothing more. Diving deep into the topic could be a whole new book, but it is important that you know that it will end. Life will get better for you or your partner. You will bond with your baby and finally feel like the mother you were born to be. It is a common and totally treatable condition, and it will pass. Therapy, rest, self-care, and medication may all be used to put you back on your way to happiness.

Being prone to depression, having a stressful pregnancy, financial problems, having a troubled relationship with those close to you and many other factors can put you at risk. If you are in danger of developing postpartum depression, talk to your doctor so that you can come up with a plan to fight it preemptively.

Cost of Having a Baby

Have you ever wondered about the price of delivering a baby? Should you live in the United States, the short answer is *a lot*. Prices vary depending on which state you live in. The least expensive childbirth occurs in Alabama, where, with insurance, delivering a child costs four thousand dollars. Without insurance, the price rises to almost ten thousand. The average cost of birth in America is ten thousand dollars; this dollar amount raises quickly the moment any complications occur. These are only the labor and delivery totals.

Almost half of all new parents underestimate the price of the first year of a baby's life. If we include the costs of the first year of life within the cost of having the baby, the price jumps from

ten thousand to twenty-three thousand. There is
no real price tag to place on the wholeness that a
child can offer to the lives of the parents.
Childbirth begins the most rewarding,
endearing, and challenging chapter in any new
mother's life.

Chapter 3: Just Baby

New mothers are tough. They are able to push through some of the some physically trying experiences. Pregnancy, labor, and delivery are all a testament to the love that a mother feels for her little one. Blood and tears are only accessories to a chaotic struggle that culminates in the creation of human life. Exhausted, she holds that newborn and smiles, knowing that all the struggle has been made worth it. In this chapter, we will take a closer look at pregnancy and delivery.

Preparation and Pregnancy (Before the Baby)

Pregnancy Tests

There is a pregnancy hormone called HCG that is only present in a women's urine if she is carrying a child. The presence of this hormone is the marker that over the counter pregnancy tests are checking for. HCG takes weeks to develop within the body, meaning that pregnancy tests cannot immediately detect the hormone at the moment of conception. Women who suspect that they're pregnant may test two weeks after their last sexual encounter or one week after a missed period.

What is a Doula?

Doulas are paid, pregnancy companions. They are trained but not medically licensed. The Doula's job is to provide support and advice to the pregnant woman and her partner.

There is scientific evidence that having a doula present during delivery can both speed up labor by twenty-five percent and reduce the need for cesarean sections by fifty percent. It's very important that an expecting mother feel supported and encouraged through her pregnancy. Female companionship can play a vital role in improving both confidence and feelings of security.

Lamaze Classes

The nature of Lamaze has been evolving and changing with the needs of pregnant women. The class aims to strengthen the confidence of pregnant women so that they are able to pass through the birthing process with less resistance. In the movies, Lamaze is represented as being mostly about controlled breathing; it is much more involved than that.
Lamaze places importance on techniques to physically and psychologically make delivery less painful. In the class, pregnant women learn about the ways that movement and relaxation

techniques can improve their experience. There are six core principals to the class:

1. Do not force the labor to start before the body is ready. Your body knows when you're ready and it should happen naturally.
2. Move throughout the process of labor. Changing positions is important; walking around is also encouraged.
3. Have a person you trust (doula, partner, family or friend) on-hand to support you through the labor.
4. Do not allow interventions with the labor, that are not a medical necessity.
5. Listen to the natural rhythm of your body, it knows when to push. Avoid birthing the child while laying on your back.
6. Do your best to stay with your baby after the labor, unless medically necessary to be separated.

Predicting Gender

As far back as human history goes, there have been wives' tales about predicting the gender of an unborn child. There are medical tests that can accurately read the gender within seven weeks of conception through DNA. Amniocentesis is also able to unveil the gender, but that procedure is more dangerous and should not be used for gender alone (we will cover this in its' own section).

Some of the more fun (but not accurate or true at all) examples of gender reading include examining the way that a mother carries her child. If the baby sits higher on the mother's abdomen, that is indicative of the child being a girl; lower is a boy. Another myth suggests that a narrow and round stomach suggests male and a less contained mass means female.

One last fun and untrue method: Take a ring that you own and tie it to a string. Lie down on the floor and hold the string (with attached ring) over your stomach. If the ring rotates, that means that you will have a girl. Swinging back and forth is indicative of a boy. Science and medicine are, of course, the only real means of finding out the gender.

Morning Sickness

Morning sickness is a term used to refer to nausea and vomiting that is associated with pregnancy. It is not specific to the morning and is very common, affecting more than half of all pregnant women. These symptoms are worst from the fourth to sixteenth week of pregnancy, most women will notice a drop off after the twelfth week.

Combating morning sickness can be done by eating and drinking small amounts during the day. Rest can also help with these symptoms. Avoid heat and close proximity to strong smells, perhaps imploring a partner to prepare your meals. Smell lemons when you feel nausea coming on. Salty snacks can also be a deterrent.

Feeling as though morning sickness has progressed past its usual deadline can be the result of the uterus pushing into the stomach of a pregnant lady. Symptoms can stick around until the third trimester. This is another instance in which limiting the portion sizes and increasing the number of times that you eat can come in handy.

Amniotic Fluid

Amniotic fluid resides inside the amniotic sac. This is a membranous "bag" that serves to protect the infant; it also has a large role in the passing of nutrients from mother to baby. This liquid also serves to keep the fetus warm while acting as the baby's supply of hormones. It offers the baby a water-like resistance to move around in so that developing muscles can gain strength. Amniotic fluid also aids in developing the fetus's lungs.

When a pregnant woman's "water breaks", it is
the rupturing of this amniotic sac. The substance
inside the sac is a clear or pale-yellow liquid that
has no smell. From thirty-six weeks of pregnancy
(at one quart of liquid), the woman will begin to
lose fluid until the delivery, when the sac is
broken.

Amniocentesis is a medical procedure in
which a hollow needle is inserted into a pregnant
woman's uterus. This allows doctors to retrieve a
sample from the amniotic sac so that they are
able to study the chromosomal make-up of the
child. This can inform of any abnormalities,
including (but not limited to): **down
syndrome, cystic fibrosis and muscular
dystrophy.** The procedure can also be used to
check for infection, lung maturity, and a
confirmation of paternity.

There is a small chance that the mother could
miscarry because of this procedure. The danger
associated with amniocentesis means that
mothers are not subjected to the testing unless
she has a genetically high risk of birth defects,
has already had a child with birth defects, or has
a concerning genetic test or lab screening.
The risk of miscarriage from the procedure is
very small. It ranges from one out of every two
hundred to one out of every four hundred. This
danger is tied to accidental induction of labor,
infection, and breaking of water.

Low Amniotic Fluid
Eight percent of pregnant women experience low amniotic fluid levels. A condition called oligohydramnios. This is most likely to occur during the third trimester. Passing a due date can cause amniotic fluid levels to drop.

The causes of oligohydramnios can vary, but the condition is often due to length of pregnancy, birth defects, leaking or punctured membrane, issues with the placenta, or dehydration of the mother. The later in the pregnancy that the lowered levels occur, the less serious the condition is. During the first four and a half months, there is a risk of miscarriage, stillbirth or compressed fetal organs. In the latter half of the pregnancy, there is a danger of pre-term birth and complications that may lead to a c-section delivery.

Preterm Birth

Preterm birth occurs when factors associated with the pregnancy necessitate that the baby is born before the forty-week gestation period is over. Babies that are born too soon can experience issues with their lungs, brain or liver, as these are the last organs to mature. There may also be issues with feeding, low weight, and slow weight gain. The immature lungs can present problems with breathing. Hearing and visual issues are also possible. The baby also has a chance of having a developmental delay or **cerebral palsy**. If at all possible, it is best for the pregnancy to reach at least thirty-nine weeks in order to avoid the risks associated with pre-term labor.

 It is important to remember that these risks are a worst-case scenario. Quitting alcohol, smoking and substance abuse can greatly reduce the chances that your child will be born prematurely. The warning signs that a pregnant woman is going to deliver prematurely are, unfortunately, just the same symptoms of labor.

When to Call a Doctor

It is important to seek medical attention for issues during the pregnancy. Even if you're the type who would rather let issues resolve on their own. Sometimes our bodies communicate larger problems through smaller problems. This is not to say that you should be stressing out or paranoid over every ailment. It's better to take precautions when it isn't a huge deal for the sake of your mental health and the wellbeing of your little one.

Moderate or heavy vaginal bleeding is at the top of this list. Twenty percent of pregnant women experience spotting within the first trimester, the flow is normally much lighter than a period. A little blood is completely normal. In the earlier trimesters, it is important to get a heavy flow checked out by a doctor to ensure that you're not experiencing an ectopic pregnancy. In later trimesters, it could be a sign that there is a complication. Bleeding alongside pain, fever, or chills is especially important to report to your doctor.

Pain in your pelvic region that lasts for days or is intense, should be reported to your healthcare provider. Vomiting that shows up alongside pain is also a good reason to call. Swelling in hands and face (especially in the later trimesters) warrants immediate attention. Swelling in the legs and feet is normal unless the foot swelling is sudden. Intense headaches or headaches that persist can indicate a larger issue, especially if they are causing dizziness. Fainting and blurred vision can also be a sign that you should call your doctor.

4-D Ultrasound

4-D ultrasound imaging is growing in popularity because it allows you to see your developing baby in incredible detail. 2-D ultrasounds are moving pictures in black and white that allow you to see a very distorted view of the fetus. These are the pocket-sized pictures that parents in the movies often show to their friends. Detail is lost in the x-ray like quality.

3-D ultrasound is a frozen image that allows the parent to get a much more dimensional look at their baby. You're able to make out details and even grasp the little one's facial expression. It's the first topographic picture that most people see of their infant.

4-D ultrasound is similar to 3-D, but it is a video instead of a still picture. It allows the parent to see their little one brought to life before their eyes. Never before have parents been allowed to take such a scared glance inside the womb.

Labor and After

Due Date

The date that a mother is given for their child's birth is just an estimation. Around five percent of babies are even born on the date that they are due. Being pregnant on or after your due date should not worry about an expecting mother. That day is only the doctors best guess based on the information provided. Accurately dating a fetus can be difficult because knowing the moment of conception may be made murky by mistaken menstrual cycles.

Most babies (eighty percent) arrive in a window of time between thirty-eight weeks and forty-two weeks. Babies aren't even considered overdue until after week forty-two, and only ten percent are born after that week. Complications associated with being overdue are rare but include the amniotic fluid running low, the baby getting too big, and the placenta running out of nutrients. The doctors will closely monitor a pregnancy that passes forty weeks, most likely with the intention to induce labor during week forty-one.

The odds are likely that you will deliver before you must be induced, with half of all women giving birth by forty weeks. Seventy-five to eighty percent through week forty-one to week forty-two.

Inducing Labor

Induction is a means by which doctors can medically stimulate the body to give birth and it can occur for a few reasons. A medical emergency can encourage doctors to induce or the choice of the mother. It can also be done when going into labor would benefit the mother or the child; more than it would be a risk. Lamaze teaches against induction, and the American College of Obstetricians and Gynecologists warns that it should only be used as a last resort.

Extended pregnancy, infection, premature rupture of the amniotic sac, nutrient-deprived placenta, and complications can all make induction medically necessary to the safety of the mother and the baby. Nipple stimulation can be used as a natural method for inducing labor by simulating a nursing child. Oxytocin is released from the brain, which is responsible for contractions. Doctors may also create a tear in the membranes around the amniotic sac, simulate contractions, or allow the pregnant mother to take an oxytocin pill. Cervical ripening may also be used, where the cervix is encouraged to open via a topical ointment or with medical devices (such as balloons or catheters).

Braxton Hicks and Labor Contractions

From time to time, you will hear women talk about false labor. When expecting mothers to experience these faux cramps, it can be uncomfortable and disorienting. Braxton Hicks contractions are a tightening and loosening of the abdominal muscles. They do not grow in intensity or duration and feel a bit like the nagging cramps that come along with menstruation.

These cramps are totally normal and are not nearly as painful as the contractions from true labor. Braxton Hicks may appear at the end of the second trimester and last into the third. This nuisance may be vanquished by walking around, as they do not seem to be able to withstand movement or switching positions. If they should occur after exercise, rest and relaxation is the answer. A nice warm bath can also be used to combat these fake contractions.

Pregnant women may also experience another sharp pain on the sides of their stomachs. **Round ligament pain** is caused by the overextension of the ligaments that hold the uterus while being attached to the pelvis. Any movement of the stomach muscles can trigger this dagger-like ache; sneezing and coughing are the enemies. The good news is that it can , using the same methods that you would for Braxton Hicks.

With all this talk of pain, we must cover actual **labor contractions**. The winding and releasing of uterine muscle fibers are responsible for this beast of a sensation that all pregnant women fear. The contractions from true pregnancy grow in intensity and duration. A woman suffering from labor contractions will notice that her stomach becomes hard during the spasm but will relax in between assaults.

Labor contractions are felt first in the lower back and migrate to the abdomen. These cramps can be used to assess how far along into your labor you are, and if you should go to the hospital. When counting contractions, get a pen and piece of paper to record the exact time that a contraction begins and ends. This will allow you to better count the time in between them and the duration of the cramp itself. When they last for almost a minute and occur less than five minutes apart, it is time to go to the hospital.

Pain Relief

The word **epidural** is famous. Some mothers swear by it, and others work to avoid it at all costs. This method of pain relief is requested and used by more than fifty percent of pregnant women. Epidurals work to block the nerve impulses from the lowest part of the spinal column. These drastically reduce all sensation in the lower body.

Epidurals are administered via a hollow needle to an area around the spinal cord. A tube is then inserted into the needle, and the needle is removed, leaving the small tube embedded in the skin. A catheter is then attached to the exposed tube so that it doesn't move around and the medicine may be dispersed to the patient, as needed.

Epidurals offer many benefits to the laboring mothers, including greatly reducing the pain involved. The medicine also allows the patient to remain conscious and aware during the birthing process. Epidurals can also be used to relax the mother and even offer the ability to rest and sleep during prolonged labor.

The downside of epidurals is mostly the consequence of the medication being shot into the spine. Permanent nerve damage is rare but possible. There is also a small chance that the patient could develop an intense headache from leaking spinal fluid, but this can be fixed. Epidurals may drop your blood pressure dramatically. Your ears might ring. Once administered, you must switch positions continuously (after a set amount of time), because laying toward one side for too long can bring the labor to a halt or greatly slow the process down. A less intense side effect of an epidural is the inability to feel yourself push and sometimes the inability to push.

Cesarean Section

A cesarean section (or c-section), it when the baby is delivered surgically from an incision in the mother's abdomen and womb. C-sections are used when there is a complicating factor in the pregnancy that increases the risk of vaginal birth, or because a mother elects for the procedure to be done. Due to the surgical nature of this method, it can take much longer to heal than a vaginal birth does. The mother will be in the hospital for three to four additional days, and the actual healing will take somewhere around six weeks. During emergency c-sections, doctors are able to deliver babies in less than twenty

minutes. Fifteen minutes of that time is the
incision.

The risks involved with getting a c-section are
the same as undergoing any surgery. There is a
chance that you could acquire an infection.
Blood clots and hemorrhages are a danger. The
patient could have a reaction to the anesthesia. A
risk that is unique to labor is that the procedure
can increase your chances of complications
during future pregnancies.

Cord Blood Storage

Cord "blood" comes from the umbilical cord
after the baby has been delivered. The term can
be deceptive because what is left in the umbilical
cord is mostly stem cells. There have been major
medical advancements as far as stem cell
research is concerned.

The cells are collected and cryogenically frozen
in a "bank" that is made for such storage. Should
a serious medical issue arise within the family,
these cells may be used to treat the illness. Some
cancers have even been treated with the
harvested cells.

The FDA has approved the treatment of more
than eighty different ailments with the stem
cells, and that number is on the rise. These cells
could eventually be used to treat autism and

cerebral palsy. With the medical benefit of harvesting stem cells, it is surprising that the cost is accessible. The initial cost of collection and preservation is one thousand to two-thousand dollars, with a fee of one to two-hundred dollars a year.

Cord Clamping

When the baby is born and the umbilical cord is still attached to the placenta, the cord is clamped on both of its furthest ends. This allows for the famous cut to be made in the middle, which separates the baby from its mother. The doctor will normally allow the partner to do the honors. An effort is also made to hold the baby near the placenta so that gravity will encourage more blood flow. There is no evidence that gravity produces any change in the amount of blood that a newborn receives, but there is a practice that allows the infant to take in more of its mother's vital blood.

Delayed cord clamping is exactly what it sounds like. The umbilical cord is traditionally clamped right after birth, but some parents are electing to wait for an additional one to three minutes before allowing the cord to be clamped. It was believed that clamping quickly would stop the mothers from losing unnecessary amounts of blood. This practice of waiting allows more blood to flow to the newborn. This can be especially important for babies that are born pre-term.

Alternatives

Homebirth is a taboo topic that we don't hear much about within the pregnancy discussion. It is completely legal in all U.S states to have an unassisted birth at one's own residence. Some areas require that a doctor's appointment be made immediately following the birth. It is, however, important to keep in mind that almost half of home pregnancies are transferred to a hospital.

This method of birth can actually be a welcome idea for women that are forecasted to have a healthy pregnancy that does not carry any added risks. Especially if the mother has elected to experience natural birth, free of medication. This option would allow the mother to deliver her baby in the comfort of her own home, surrounded by family and loved ones. Homebirth enables the laborer to have much more freedom and peace of mind.

Midwives/nurses make the perfect addition to this process and allow the benefit of having a medical professional present. The presence of a doula would also be incredibly beneficial to the mother. Home pregnancies are about sixty percent less expensive than at a hospital, which could mean four thousand dollars, instead of six thousand.

Water Birth is another alternative to traditional labor. It is centered around the idea that a warm tub will be a more familiar environment for the baby to arrive it. It is easier for the baby to exit the womb and less trying for the mother.
Waterbirth must always be under the advice and supervision of a medical professional. This is a great option for home birth under a midwife's watchful eye, but many hospitals and birthing centers are also working to accommodate mothers who desire a water birth. If you are interested in trying water birth, it is worth the call to your hospital of choice.

The benefits include the ease of changing positions and moving around because of the buoyancy of water. The weightless feeling also works to remove the stress off of a mother's body. Water can also cause the skin to become slightly more elastic, meaning that tearing is also reduced. Waterbirth has the added benefit of making the mother feel more at ease due to increased privacy offered by the tub.

No matter which method of delivery you happen to choose, the result will be safe. Through the tears and sweat, you will meet the eyes of a tiny human who will change the way that you love forever. Congratulations on this journey, and I hope that it is everything you are hoping for and more.

Conclusion

Thank you for reading through to the end of *My First Pregnancy: Information, Advice, and Tips for New Parents*. I hope that this book has been able to shine a helpful light on the process of pregnancy and childbirth. This book was created with the intention of providing information to expecting mothers in a relatable and casual way.

The chapters in this book were written with you in mind. I wanted to create an interesting and fun way to gain answers to all of the most asked questions in relation to being a brand new mom. I want this to be a resource that you can return to time and time again. I've endeavored to include all the essentials within these pages and even a few passages that are crafted in the spirit of pure entertainment.

Pregnancy is one of the most astounding processes that the human body is capable of. It is the furthering of our species and the creation of the next generation. Carrying a child is the closest thing to actual magic. It's also difficult, painful, stressful, and brave. The bond between a mother and her infant is a power that nothing else may touch. I hope that this book has helped you prepare for this impressive task. I would also like to say congratulations and the best of luck to you in this new chapter in your life.

Additionally, if you enjoyed or found use out of this book, please take a moment to leave a review on Amazon.

www.ingramcontent.com/pod-product-compliance
Lightning Source LLC
Chambersburg PA
CBHW070757250726
48662CB00004B/1843